Beauty Secrets for Older Women

How to look Young and Stay Beautiful

Katherine P. Rose

Table of Contents

Introduction

At some point, you've probably heard or felt that after a certain age you should throw on a housecoat and a pair of slippers, settle in front of the television with a cup of tea, and not care about how you look anymore. You think that at this age it doesn't matter what you wear, how you look, what you do, or how you feel.

Repeat after me: You are never too old to look and feel beautiful!

It doesn't matter if you're 20, 50, 70, or even 90. Every woman deserves to look and feel their very best at every stage in their life! This isn't to say that it's always going to be easy to do, especially if you have a partner, family, job, home, and/or various other responsibilities. However, it's absolutely doable if you're committed to the process. It takes preparation, hard work, and effort; but the results are worth it. Sometimes, even starting with one small change can alter your life for the better.

Beauty isn't just about makeup tips and how you do your hair; it's also about carrying yourself and feeling what you wear. "Beauty Secrets for Older Women" doesn't just discuss what type of makeup you should use or how to do your hair in a flattering way... this book will also discuss the many aspects of how to look and feel your best from head-to-toe from the time to change your wardrobe to building your self confidence. Just remember that it's never too late to make positive changes.

Going back to the 'let it all go after a certain age' mentality, many beauty books are geared toward women in their 20s and 30s as if you shouldn't even bother to try anymore after a certain age. However, that's far from the case. Let this book be proof that you can look and feel fabulous from the inside out at any age.

With that said, it's time to settle in and get started on discussing some of the best beauty secrets for older women.

CHAPTER 2
It's All in the Attitude

There's a reason so many people say that confidence is everything. Your attitude can make or break how beautiful you are; it doesn't matter where you are on the looks scale. When you have a great personality, you're instantly more attractive.

Improving your attitude isn't only better for you, but also for your relationships. Think about it: would you rather spend time with someone who is drop-dead gorgeous with an ugly personality, or someone is average but an absolute winner in the personality department?

When you feel good about yourself and have a great attitude, you shine from the inside out. At some point, you've probably spent time around someone who didn't have a high confidence level or had a negative attitude towards life; maybe even both. Chances are their energy was low, their presence was draining on you, and they didn't have light in their eyes. When someone radiates happiness and confidence, you gravitate toward them because you subconsciously want to feel the way they do.

It doesn't matter how old you are; keeping a high confidence level is important. So how exactly do you go about building a positive attitude?

Improving Your Confidence

Get a makeover

Sometimes all you need is to give yourself a makeover to kick your confidence up a notch. Even something as simple as buying a new outfit, changing your makeup style, or getting a haircut can make you feel better about yourself.

Do things you've always wanted to

Whether you want to get a college degree or go skydiving, you can do whatever you want, regardless of age. When you start checking things off your bucket list, you're going to feel better about yourself overall. Achieving your goals can be a great confidence builder.

Give back to others

It's amazing how great you can feel about yourself just by giving back to others, and you don't need a lot of money to do it. Baking cookies for a neighbor, volunteering your time, or putting a love note in your partner's jacket pocket can give you an instant boost.

Stop comparing yourself to others

One of the greatest things about living on a planet with more than 7 billion people is that no two individuals are the same. You never know what's going on in someone else's life, so while you're kicking yourself for not having a marriage like your neighbor has, you may not realize that they're headed for divorce. Or maybe you wish you could look like your 50-year-old model cousin when she's secretly envious of your success. Rather than focusing on what you don't have or what you think others have, concentrate on everything good about yourself and your life.

Exercise

Not only does exercising give you a mood-booster from the endorphins, but your body will start to look better, and in turn, improve your confidence. If you hate working out, try something that doesn't seem like exercise such as walking your dog more often. Every week or so, start increasing how much you do this.

Developing a Positive Attitude

Focus on the positive

There's always going to be negative situations that come up in life, but when you handle them positively, it's typically easier to deal with. Try to make the best of every situation, even if you have to force yourself at first. Once you start, it will gradually become a habit.

Realize you can't control everything

Let's say you're on the way home from work and you're excited about an evening of sitting on the couch and watching a movie, when you suddenly hit a massive traffic jam. This is one of those situations you can't change. Short of your car suddenly sprouting wings or the cars parting so you can drive through, you don't have much of a choice but just riding it out. Getting upset is essentially pointless, and all you're going to accomplish is making yourself miserable. Rather than throwing a fit, blast some music in your car and sing. Make your own fun and make the best of what's going on so any situation can be better.

Think positive without expectations

How many times have you thought that by simply thinking positively you would somehow force the universe to give you what you want? However, if this doesn't happen, the negativity can build up and your positivity will sink. Sure, a little disappointment is natural, but having expectations that you're going to get something simply because you have a positive mindset will set you up for severe disappointment if it doesn't happen. Always think about the best without expecting it to happen so it's a wonderful surprise.

Laugh a little

Yes, life can be rough... but it's incredible how much laughing can change things for the better. Life usually isn't as big of a deal as we make it out to be, and you can just think: How serious is it in the grand scheme of things? Life is often only as serious as we make it, so laugh a little!

Building up your confidence and developing a positive attitude are two separate things, but they often tie together. So when you start working on one, you're automatically working on the other. Just remember: it doesn't matter what age you are; you can always improve your confidence and attitude for the better. It will make you more beautiful than you can imagine!

CHAPTER 3
Your Old Routine Isn't Working

Let's talk about two of the worst habits older women have when it comes to beauty:

They don't change their beauty habits as they get older.
They keep their makeup routine the same as when they were younger.

I'll give you a minute to think about the last time you changed your makeup style or your beauty habits. It's probably been awhile, right? Keeping the same routine and using the same makeup typically doesn't constitute as a 'tried and true' method, but instead can make you look older than you actually are. Most women age themselves and don't even realize it. Could you be one of them?

The Lifespan of Makeup

You can keep unopened makeup for years, but once you open it and the air hits, the clock starts ticking and it begins to degrade. Chances are, you're not going to remember when you bought each product and opened it. Save yourself the hassle by purchasing small neon green dot stickers, writing the expiration date on each one for when to toss it, and slapping them on each individual piece of makeup.

So what exactly is the lifespan on beauty products?

Mascara – You should either toss mascara once every three months or when it becomes clumpy, whichever happens first. Mascara is dark and wet, so it's the perfect place for bacteria to grow. Keep it too long and you're essentially putting a glob of bacteria on your eye every time you apply.

Eye shadow and eyeliner – Powdered eye shadow can stay for two years while cream eyeshadows should be tossed after six months. Pencil eyeliners can last up to two years, but just like liquid eyeliners, you should toss them after three months so you don't put yourself at risk for an infection with every use.

Nail polish – You can keep nail polish for one to two years, or until it dries out or gets clumpy; whichever happens first.

Lipstick, lip liner, and lip gloss – A lip liner is good for two years. Lipsticks and lip gloss can be kept up to two years or if they dry out; whichever happens first.

Skin products – Check for expiration date sand go by that, but if it doesn't have one, toss it after six months.

Powder face makeup and liquid face makeup – You can keep powders for two years, but toss liquid face makeup after three months.

Sunscreen – Check for an expiration date. They typically last around one year.

Changing Your Beauty Habits

Every few years or so, it's a good idea to reevaluate your overall appearance and make tweaks here and there. You can continue to do the same beauty routine you did when you were 20, but it's not going to do much for you as you get older. Here are some beauty habits to consider changing and incorporating into your routine, if you haven't done so already.

Drink more water – As you get older, your skin tends to dry out. Water is great for your body, and it's going to help make your skin look amazing.

Change your makeup style – When you were younger, you might have pulled off liquid eyeliner and dark lipstick fabulously. However, it's different when you get older. Certain pieces and colors of makeup are now more of a detriment to your look than an enhancement. Soften your makeup and you'll be surprised by the results.

Get more sleep – Years ago, you may have been able to get by with only four hours of sleep a night. However, getting seven or eight hours can not only help you feel more refreshed, it can give your body a chance to restore itself. It can also help prevent those pesky dark under-eye circles.

Use a humidifier – As previously stated, your skin dries out as you get older. Using a humidifier every night can help incorporate more moisture into your skin.

Flossing – Many of those who are younger tend to blow off flossing, but it's a habit that's better started sooner than later. If you don't floss yet, consider all the reasons why you should. Not only is it much more effective than just brushing, it can help prevent periodontal disease, which is a contributing factor to heart disease and diabetes. Not to mention a piece of spinach in your teeth is never an attractive look!

Moisturize more often – If you haven't been moisturizing your skin for years, you're already behind... but that doesn't mean it's too late! Moisturize twice per day (once in the morning and once right before bed) all over your body. You will drastically improve the look, feel, and condition of your skin.

Use anti-aging products – There are many who put off using anti-aging products because they think it's a sign they're getting old, but frankly, it's just smart to use them. Let's face it, we're all getting older... but using anti-aging products can help reverse the signs of aging and improve your look. The sooner you use them, the better. Look for products that contain Pentapeptides, which reportedly helps stimulate collagen growth and encourages the skin to repair itself.

Meditate – Stress can severely age you, so when you take the time to relax and calm your mind at least once or twice a day, it will do wonders for how you look and feel. Meditation can be a great thing, and the best part is that you can do it anywhere from your bedroom to the bathroom at work. If all you have is a few minutes, it can still do wonders.

All of the above mentioned may seem too tiring and require time and effort, but they will become more of a habit than a hassle. The rewards are very much worth it! Get started on the positive changes today and you may be surprised just how quickly you start to look and feel more beautiful.

Chapter 4
Finding Your Passion

You may remember the "let it go after a certain age" mentality that I mentioned in the introduction, where many think that once you hit a certain age, you should essentially sit in front of the television all day and not too much of anything. How wrong they are.

When you're getting older is the best time to find your passion, develop new hobbies, learn new things, etc. Not only do you now have more money to pursue what you want to do, but you are also more in tune with what you like and don't like. Chances are, you're also at an age where you couldn't care less about people's opinions or what they think of you, so you're also short of fear in that regard. The only think that's probably stopping you is your excuses.

One of the biggest excuses many people make as they get older is that they're "too old" to try something new: they're too old to get their college degree, they're too old to test out that sports car, they're too old to go skydiving, they're too old to take a cooking class, etc. That excuse is a waste of time, energy, and life. That's like saying that younger people shouldn't crochet, scrapbook, or garden because they're "too young." It sounds pretty silly when you reverse the stereotypes, doesn't it? Saying you're "too old" sounds the exact same way.

Do you really want to pass up on an exciting and fulfilling experience because of two little numbers? Your age doesn't dictate what you're about, you do, and taking risks, improving your knowledge, and having passion can make you downright beautiful, not to mention it improves your confidence and builds your brainpower.

There are a plethora of things you can do, but here are just some of the many, many hobbies that are great for anyone of any age to try:

Painting
Wine/beer making
Learning an instrument
Putting together model kits
Cycling
Bowling

Photography
Cake/cupcake decorating
Fishing
Taking cooking classes
Reading
Genealogy

Camping

Reef keeping

Hiking

Woodworking

Writing

Jewelry making

Learning card games

Learning a language

Restoration

Swimming

Crocheting

Scrapbooking

Volunteering

Gardening

Taking dance classes

Furthering your education

Golfing

Yoga

Traveling

Spending time with a pet

With so many options, and so much life to live, there's no reason you should feel like you have to sit around the house and do nothing. Let others waste their life or tell you that you're "too old" while you're out enjoying yourself and having a great time. It's a big world with so much to do and see, and still so much happiness to have. So go out and get to it!

CHAPTER 5
Common Beauty Mistakes Made By Older Women

As women get older, many tend to make beauty mistakes that age them, and some can't understand what they're doing wrong. Then there are those who don't even realize that they can look years younger than they currently do, and all it would take is a few changes to their makeup routine. Keep on reading for some of the most common beauty mistakes that are made by older women.

Piling on the makeup

There are some who think that piling on the foundation, eye shadow, and lipstick is going to make them look younger when it completely has the opposite effect. When it comes to makeup, you should always look like you're barely wearing any. Your face is a blank slate, and covering it up too much only hides its natural beauty.

Using bad foundation

Referring to foundation as "bad" can mean four things: it's too old, it doesn't match your complexion, it's not blended correctly, or you're using one that's not compatible with your face. After three months, it's time to replace your current foundation and buy a new one. Also, choose a foundation color that's right for your skin tone, and if you're not sure what that is, head over to a makeup counter at a department store and they'll be able to help you. After you apply it, you should make sure to blend it correctly, especially at your hairline, jaw line, and by your ears. Lastly, even if you get the color right, it doesn't mean the foundation is going to be good for your face. For example, you might need one that's specially made for dry skin. Always spot test first before committing and putting it all over your face.

Not using primer

As you get older, your skin dries out and lines and creases start to form, so when you put makeup on, it often settles into all those little areas and can make the makeup look caked on rather than smooth. Apply a primer first so you have a smooth surface to work with every time.

Not moisturizing

I've already said numerous times how important it is to moisturize, and you'll probably hear me say it at least a couple more, but one of the biggest mistakes many older women make is that they don't moisturize enough. Considering how skin can dry out through the aging process, it's vital that you continue to keep it hydrated so it looks its best.

Sporting thin brows

The thinner the eyebrows, the older you'll look. Eyebrows already thin out with age, so if you pluck them thinking it's making it better, it's not. Fill them in with a powder that's slightly lighter than your brow color, and start getting your eyebrows professionally done.

Going for bright makeup

Have you ever seen older women who are wearing bright blue eye shadow up to their eyebrows or have neon pink eyeliner lining their lids? It's not an attractive look, and it's not hard to wonder where they're going like that. Leave the bright makeup colors to those who are 21 and headed to a nightclub.

Not changing your makeup routine

Different ages call for a different beauty routine, but many women are still sporting the same look they did when they were two decades younger. Make sure your makeup is right for your age and skin tone and you'll look younger in minutes.

Wearing dark lipstick

Wearing a dark lipstick makes your mouth look smaller, and combined with the fact that our lips thin as we get older; it makes for an unattractive look. Stick to a lighter shade for a fuller looking pout.

Doing too much lip liner

Lip liner is meant to do just that – line the lips – it's not supposed to be the only thing on your lips and it's not even supposed to be noticeable. Draw a thin line and make sure that it's completely blended with your lipstick or lip gloss.

If you find that you've been making some of the aforementioned mistakes, don't worry about it. The great thing about makeup is that you can switch it out in minutes and it can give you a completely different look. A few changes here and there can have you looking younger than you have in years.

CHAPTER 6
Not all Hype is Good Hype

When it comes to beauty, there's always something different coming out in the media that promises you'll look younger in minutes or drop weight fast... but that's not always the case. Sure, there are great products that do fantastic things, but between makeup, surgery, diets, and other products, the amount that are making promises they can't keep is enough to make your head spin, and quite a few of them aren't going to give you the results you're hoping for.

As an example, let's just look at a list of some of the more "unique" diet fads that have been around and developed a following. Some work, some don't, but either way they're certainly not the diets you're probably used to.

Twinkie diet – Eating only Twinkies for meals with Doritos as a snack

Cigarette diet – Stemming from the 1920s, companies promoted smoking rather than reaching for junk food.

Breatharian diet – There's been two versions that I've seen. One is that you hold the food up to your mouth and breathe it in, but don't take a bite. Another version states that you don't even have to do that, that breathing the air alone is enough.

Baby food diet – Baby food replaces one or two meals a day, and the third meal is healthy and balanced.

Cookie diet – You eat specially made cookies for breakfast, lunch, and snacks, and have a healthy balanced meal for dinner.

Hard-boiled egg diet – Eggs for breakfast, eggs for lunch, and eggs for dinner. That's it.

Tapeworm diet – You swallow a beef tapeworm that comes in pill form, and it sits in your intestines and eats any food you swallow.

Cotton ball diet – You dip four or five cotton balls in a smoothie or orange juice, and then swallow them.

Master Cleanse Diet – Drink a mix of water, cayenne pepper, lemon juice, and maple syrup.

It should go without saying, but there's no way you should try a new diet without consulting with a doctor and/or a nutritionist, especially if you have a medical condition. Some diets like the tapeworm diet or the cotton ball diet should not be tried at all. Certain diets, like the baby food diet and the Master Cleanse Diet, may work, but it's up to the doctor and/or nutritionists to give their okay on the matter before you proceed.

The aforementioned diets are just a touch of some of the diet and beauty fads that are out there that encourage people to try strange things in an effort to look young, lose weight, or look more beautiful, but the fact of the matter is a lot of things that are out there are just empty promises. The easy way isn't always the best way, and many have become sick, injured, or even died trying to achieve perfection.

When it comes to putting something on or in your body, you should always do extensive research. If you find something that seems like a great idea, but there are so many warnings out there and your gut is telling you something isn't right, it's probably best to stay away from it. Should you find something that might work for you, it's not going to hurt to run it by a medical professional. If you really want to improve the feel and look of your body, stick to the tried and true methods that really work: healthy eating, exercise, great makeup, building your confidence and developing positive thinking, and if necessary, bringing in a medical professional to give you some guidance.

CHAPTER 7
The Inner and Outer Inspection

The older you get, the more important it is to stay up-to-date with health check-ups. There are many who blow them off and thin if there seems to be nothing currently wrong, it's pointless to spend the time and money for a check-up. However, there are times where something might be wrong and you just don't know it. If you get a check-up and find the problem early, it's likely to be much less costly and detrimental than if you found it at a later date.

Physicals – Get a physical once per year, and make sure your doctor checks your cholesterol levels, does a blood test, does a bone mineral density test, and does a diabetes screening.

Skin screenings – The skin is the largest organ on the body and it goes through a lot. You should always check at least once a week for something that doesn't seem right, like an oddly-shaped mole. However, visit your dermatologist once a year just to get a skin screening, especially for places you can't usually see, like your back.

Dental check-up – Get a teeth cleaning and oral exam once every six months, but if you have any tooth or gum pain, or you notice your gums are swollen and bleeding, schedule an appointment beforehand.

Mammogram – Women should typically start getting regular mammograms at age 40, but if you have a history of breast cancer in your family and you're at high risk, you can start even earlier. It's typically recommended that, after age 40, you get a mammogram annually.

Gynecological exam

Once you start having sex, you should have an annual gynecological exam. You'll get a pap test and pelvic exam as well as get tested for STDs.

The aforementioned may seem pointless if you view yourself to be at the peak of health, but if you want to stay that way, getting check-ups when you're supposed to is a great idea. If you have children, you'll also serve as an example that taking care of your body is important, even if you seem to be in excellent health.

To make sure you don't forget to schedule your exams, set them while you're already at your previous appointment. For example, if you set an appointment in December of this year, while you're leaving that appointment, set the appointment for the following year. While there's a chance you might have to change it once the date gets much closer, at least you'll know you're due and the office can follow-up and reschedule you.

CHAPTER 8
Beverages and Your Body

The beverages you put in your body are just as important as what you eat. They can have an effect on everything from your weight to how you feel, even how your health progresses over the years. Let's take a look at five of the most common drinks people have on a daily basis.

Water

Drinking water can be hugely beneficial for your health as well as your body, and as I've already mentioned before, water can help your skin look healthy and smooth rather than dry and dull. Some of the other reported benefits of drinking water include that it helps you boost your immunity, can help you increase your energy levels, flushes out toxins from the body, and can help you lose weight as it helps you feel more full, especially if you drink a glass before your meal and while you're eating.

Wine

There are pros and cons of drinking wine, and before we get to the positives, let's talk about the cons, which can include causing additional acidity in the body, contributing to migraines, and adding up in calories. The amount of calories varies from type to type, but typically the average count is 123 calories per serving. There are also several benefits that have reportedly been found from drinking wine, including lowering the risk of heart disease, stroke, and diabetes.

Alcohol

Chances are you've had a hangover at some point in your life, which is already a giant downfall in itself, but drinking too much alcohol can have a very negative long term effect on the body as well. For example, it can be responsible for damaging the liver, heart, and pancreas, as well as causing brain problems and increasing your chances of developing cancer. It may also temporarily weaken your immune system.

Caffeine

More than half of Americans drink coffee on a daily basis, but depending on whom you ask it could either be good or bad. There's long been a debate over whether or not caffeine is actually good for you. Some of the downsides of drinking caffeine in the short term can include irritability, headaches, anxiousness, a fast heartbeat, and the inability to properly sleep, while positive effects can include alertness, better concentration, and increased energy levels. Some negative long term effects, especially for coffee drinkers who are older, may include an increased risk for getting high blood pressure, experiencing bone loss, and having higher cholesterol levels, while some positive long term effects could be a decreased chance of having a heart attack, getting cancer, getting diabetes, and developing Parkinson's.

Soda

There are quite a few downsides to drinking soda, especially on a daily basis. Soda can cause weight gain, might screw with your hormones, and may contribute to cancer. Additionally drinking soda may quicken the aging process, and the acidity can damage your teeth. There's not much point in using anti-aging products if you're only going to put something into your body that could age you faster.

Slowing down (or stopping) the amount of a particular beverage you drink isn't easy, but it can be worth it if it can help prevent you from developing a variety of diseases and health problems in the future, not to mention keep you from aging faster. Stick to the good-for-you beverages like water, and you might be surprised of how great you feel.

CHAPTER 9
Finding Your Foods

It's important to eat well, regardless of your age... but it's even more so the older you get. It may not seem like a big deal to revel in junk food on a daily basis, but it could have quite a negative effect on your health. A little dessert here or there isn't the problem; it's when junk becomes part of your everyday life and you're not eating properly balanced meals, it becomes an issue.

Healthy eating can have a hugely positive effect on your body, and some of the many benefits can include weight loss, a healthier and better look, increased energy, less of a chance of developing diseases, having a stronger immune system, living longer, having improved brain power, and having better digestion. Keep reading to learn more about some of the best foods you should be eating and how much of them.

Fish

Fish is a good source of vitamin D, Omega-3, proteins, and good fats. You should have 5 to 7 ounces of protein per day, so having a piece of fish, along with brown rice and vegetables, is a great option for dinner.

Beans

Beans are another great option for protein, and due to their fiber content, they're great for staying regular, preventing stomach problems, and easing constipation. If you're worried about how beans could bloat you, you can talk to your doctor about taking an over-the-counter medicine like Beano®.

Fruits and vegetables

You should have about 3 cups of vegetables per day and about 2 cups of fruit. So how can you eat more fruits and veggies? Two cups of a leafy vegetable equates to about 3 cups of cooked veggies, so you can have a big salad for lunch (and throw some tuna while you're at it) or dinner. For fruits, have a piece for breakfast, another for a snack, and then some for dessert.

Dairy

Those who are getting older need more calcium to prevent bone loss, and dairy is a great way to incorporate it into your diet. However, opt for low fat-versions. You can have an egg for breakfast, peanut butter on an apple for a snack, or have peanut butter on multi-grain bread for lunch. Have a cup of Greek yogurt with berries for dessert so you can have a little fruit thrown in as well.

Grains

Whole grains are better than refined grains, so you should always try to switch out one for the other. For example, rather than have white bread, opt for multi-grain bread or whole wheat, and rather than white rice, go for brown rice.

When you eliminate a lot of the junk in your diet, you may be surprised just how much better you feel. Even a few simple changes can improve your health and look for the better. You don't have to dive right in; start out small and work your way up to cleaning your eating habits.

CHAPTER 10
What Goes in Shows Itself

Anything you put on or in your body is eventually going to show itself on your outward appearance (as well as internally). We've already discussed the pros and cons of beverages and foods, but let's talk about one thing that can also have a major affect on your looks and how you feel: cigarettes. There are many who smoke every day or experience secondhand smoke. But do you really know what you're doing to your body?

Smoking cigarettes, especially for an extended period of time, can ruin your body, as well as your looks. The sooner you break the habit, the better! There are now more methods than ever to help you to stop.

Some effects smoking has on the body include:

- Loss of bone density
- Increases your chance of developing high blood pressure
- Causing an aneurysm
- Causing a stroke
- Causing eye problems, such as cataracts and macular degeneration.
- Causing over a dozen types of cancer, including in the lungs, stomach, bladder, kidney, lip, and rectum
- Causing cardiovascular disease
- Damaging your lungs, including causing asthma, pneumonia, emphysema, and bronchitis

In terms of the beauty aspect, smoking can cause:

- Bags to develop under the eyes
- Yellowed teeth
- Yellowed fingers and nails
- Brittle nails
- Psoriasis
- Warts

- Thinning hair
- Wrinkles
- Age spots
- Dull complexion

Yes, having a cigarette may make you feel relaxed, but it's also jam packed with more than 7,000 chemicals, and every time you take a puff, that's what you're putting into your body. In the end, if you should end up with a disease caused by all those cigarettes, is it really going to be worth it?

CHAPTER 11
Beauty and the Wardrobe

One of the best benefits of getting older is that you learn more about your style, figure out what you do and don't like, and what you're comfortable with. The latter of which can be a blessing and a curse, but more on that later.

How you dress can make a huge difference in how you feel about yourself, the energy you give off, and how you're perceived. However, there are many women who make some big mistakes in regards to fashion as they get older, which means they're not putting their best self forward. Below are some of the worst fashion crimes you can make as you're getting older that you should try to avoid at all costs.

Fashion crimes to avoid

Wearing comfy/un-stylish clothing

Not everything you wear is going to be 100 percent comfortable, but the majority of what you wear absolutely should be. However, there's plenty of comfortable clothing that is also stylish. For example, instead of going grocery shopping in an oversized, stained sweatshirt and a pair of sweats, throw on a pair of jeans and a well-fitting t-shirt.

Wearing outdated styles

There's a huge difference between vintage chic and an outdated mess. Just like your makeup, your wardrobe should frequently get evaluated. There's nothing wrong with wearing vintage or vintage-inspired clothing, but mix-and-match them with modern pieces if you're going to wear them. For example, wear a vintage dress, but pair it with modern jewelry and a pair of black pumps. On the other hand, there's also some past fashion styles, such as gold lamé, that should just be burned and completely ignored.

Wearing loose clothing

Wearing oversized and loose clothing does absolutely nothing for your figure, and it could even drag your mood down because you're not going to feel your best if you don't look your best. If the clothes are too big on you, then toss them – except for your favorite oversized hoodie you wear at home that's too amazing to throw out that you should never get rid of.

Wearing clothing that's too tight or revealing

There are some who try to regain their youth as they're getting older by wearing clothes that are too tight or revealing. Not only does this look absolutely ridiculous – and people will immediately identify that you're likely going through a mid-life crisis – but it's not projecting who you are in the best way. You can still show off your figure without showing off too much skin.

Dressing frumpy

Many women as they get older just give up on dressing well and opt for looking frumpy instead. This is simply because it's easier to do. However, putting together a great outfit doesn't take much thought or energy, and it can help you look much younger than you are.

Dressing your best

Dress for your body shape

Your body shape is everything when it comes to choosing clothing, and it all has to do with paying attention to your body and what looks best on it. For example, if you have a pear body shape, you'll want to wear pants that have a wider hem, opt for strapless dresses, go for A-line skirts, and stick to dark colored pants.

Wear your best shades

Not every color is going to look great on you. For example, yellow is one of those colors that aren't going to look fabulous on everyone. It's important to know what colors work for you and what don't, and if you need some help, ask a friend to go shopping with you and help you pick out what colors look best on you.

Get tailored

Getting your clothes tailored can mean the difference between looking frumpy and looking fantastic. Get that dress fitted to your body, get the pants hemmed, and make sure that what you're wearing perfectly suits you.

Show your style

Forget trends. They mean anything if they don't make you happy. Wear clothing that shows off your style and who you are, not what fashion forecasters are saying is going to be the next new hot thing next season (unless, of course, you actually like it).

Wear what's comfortable and stylish

As previously stated, there are plenty of clothes out there that are not only comfortable, but also stylish. You don't have to choose one over the other. It may take time to find the right pieces, but to make it easier, start with basic pieces that can get thrown into a lot of different outfits. For example, find a comfortable white well-fitting t-shirt, a black blazer, a new pair of jeans, a pair of black dress pants, a white button-down and a little black dress (LBD).

Look put together

You should always look put-together in whatever you're wearing whether it's a pair of jeans or a LBD. Brush your hair, throw on a little makeup, and make sure all your clothes are well-fitting and free of rips and stains.

Dress age appropriate

Many women have a tendency to not dress age-appropriate as they're getting older, and it doesn't necessarily mean dressing in styles that are better on a 25-year-old. I'm also referring to wearing clothing that makes women look like they're 5 or 10. Just because you're getting older doesn't mean you have to cling to the fashions of your youth or give up and dress like you don't care. Show off your style and your fabulous figure! Tock clothes that are perfectly you and your style.

Fashion is supposed to be fun, not hard work. Sure, it's going to take a little planning to revamp your wardrobe... but once you have it down, the rest will become habit. When you look great, you feel beautiful; like your best self. You shine from within, and that's what true beauty is all about.

Chapter 12
Let's Talk About Sex

Other than the feel-good aspect of having sex (and the pregnancy aspect), there are actually quite a few other benefits it can have in terms of your health, body, and beauty. Almost everyone has sex, so we might as well learn why having it – especially more often and regularly – is so beneficial.

Better sleep

Prolactin (a hormone in your body) releases when you have an orgasm, and in turn, help your mind and body relax to feel sleepier. Therefore, more sex = feeling more sleepy/relaxed = better sleep.

Improved immune system

The more sex you have, the more Immunoglobulin A (aka IgA) you'll have in your body. It's present in your saliva, so when you're building up to orgasm, you're actually building up your immune system at the same time.

Reduced pain

Having an orgasm has been known to reduce pain that stems from a variety of issues, including headaches, menstruation, arthritis, etc. The next time you're not feeling your best, instead of saying that you're not in the mood because you don't feel well, try having sex instead.

Improved bladder control

As you get older, maintaining bladder control can become a major issue, but when you have an orgasm, it strengthens your pelvic muscles because you're working them out. That could help in the short and long term better maintain bladder control.

It's a great work out

Foreplay and sex can burn quite a few calories, and it's one of those workouts that don't even seem like actual exercise. Sex itself can burn more than 140 calories within 30 minutes; however, having a hot and heavy make-out session can burn more than 230. Even if you don't want to go all out and have sex, at least have a really great make-out session instead.

Less stress

Oxytocin and endorphins, also known as your feel-good hormones, are released during sex, which can help you feel less stressed overall, especially if you're worrying about a particular situation or event.

Younger looks

More estrogen is released when you have sex, which can help you look and feel younger. Consider sex one of the best anti-aging methods there is.

Sex can help you feel happier, and that shows with an almost glow. There are very few things that can make you more beautiful than when you're happy. Try to have sex with your partner more often (initiate if you have to) and see if you notice any of the aforementioned changes. It may just inspire you and your partner to have a more active sex life!

CHAPTER 13
Anti-aging Products

As you get older, chances are anti-aging products are going to become your best friend. With so many on the market, it can be difficult to know which ones to choose. But it's vital to pick one that's going to work best for you. One product may work for many years, but your skin changes; especially as you get older. You'll likely have to switch it out for something that's more tailored to the current condition of your skin. When you're choosing an anti-aging cream, there are several things to consider when you're choosing the best one.

Price

Many women automatically go for the most expensive anti-aging product that's in the fanciest box with the most elaborate name simply because they think it's the best, but that's not always the case at all. Take a look at beauty sites and magazines who put out a list of their recommendations of the best anti-aging products, and you'll see a good mix of hi/low products. Go for what will work best for you, not for what has the highest price tag.

Your skin type

There's a slew of anti-aging products out there that are specially tailored to certain skin types. For example, you might need one for sensitive skin, dry skin, or oily skin. Before you get a product, determine first what type of skin you're working with and you can significantly narrow down your options.

Your aging concern

What are you most worried about when it comes to your skin and aging? Are you worried about wrinkles around your eyes or maybe age spots? When you're shopping around, look for the anti-aging product that treats your specific concern.

Sunscreen

Many anti-aging products contain sunscreen, but not all, and as you know, getting too much sun can cause wrinkles on your face as well as skin cancer. Opt for an anti-aging product that has at least an SPF 30 so you can product yourself from the sun's rays while you're fighting wrinkles.

Reputation

Reputation can be pretty important when it comes to buying an anti-aging product, so make sure to take that into consideration when you're shopping around. There are always going to be people who were unsatisfied with one product or another, but if that's the majority, or there were complaints about serious issues, move onto a different product.

Pentapeptides

When you're shopping for anti-aging products, look for those that contain Pentapeptides. There's research that states it can help repair skin and encourage collagen production, which can give your skin a more youthful, firmer look.

Before buying any anti-aging product, take your time and do research to find one that's right for you. If you have any questions or concerns, or you just can't seem to find the right product, consult with a reputable Esthetician who can help you pick the best one.

CHAPTER 14
The Skin You're In

The face is the forefront of who you are. One of the misconceptions many women have is that you aren't attractive if you don't have flawless features. Actually, you don't have to be a drop-dead gorgeous model to be beautiful. As previously stated, when you're happy and confident, it radiates through you, makes your skin glow, and makes your eyes shine. However, we're all born with only one face, so we might as well do what we can to keep it in the best condition possible and help it look its best. Whether it is makeup or corrective or preventative methods, there are several ways you can keep your face looking more beautiful than you ever thought possible.

Skin treatments

There are a lot of different skin treatments out there to try that could help you combat the skin's aging process. Two of the most popular options are Botox, which temporarily paralyzes the facial muscles to remove wrinkles, and Restylane, which is a filler that can plump the skin and help erase lines. Those looking to revitalize their complexion and skin tone might want to consider microdermabrasion, which is essentially an extreme exfoliation process. Chemical peels can also help, and it works by removing the top layers of your skin so when it grows back, it's smoother and more youthful. The aforementioned isn't right for everyone, especially if you have allergies or sensitive skin, so consult with a dermatologist first before proceeding.

Foundation

Foundation can even-out skin tone and can make you have a more youthful appearance, but it's not going to do anything if you don't apply it the right way or you use the wrong one. It's a must to choose one that's the right shade, blend it correctly especially around the jaw, ears, and hairline, and not continue to use one that's past the point of its prime (three months). Considering skin tends to try out as you get older, liquid foundations will be your best bet.

Blush

As you get older, your skin is going to start to lose its rosy hue in the cheeks, which means a little blush is just what you need to help bring back that youthful appearance. However, you should opt for cream blush rather than the powder blush you're used to. When lines and wrinkles form, the powder blush can just sit in there while cream goes on more smoothly.

Primer

I know, I know, you're probably thinking that your face isn't a wall and doesn't need primer. However, that's essentially what your skin is: a barrier. And almost everyone's skin has lines and bumps that can get in the way of makeup going on flawlessly! That's where primer comes in. It creates an even surface to work with so your makeup goes on better. Put it on after you apply your moisturizer.

Moisturizer

I cannot continue to emphasize enough the importance of using moisturizer. The more hydrated your skin is, the better, and the more youthful it will look. Opt for a moisturizer that has an SPF of at least 30, and make sure to choose one that's ideal for your skin type, such as one that's specifically for dry skin.

Sleep

When you get a good night's sleep – about 7 to 8 hours – your skin has a good chance to repair itself. Too little sleep, and not only do the dreaded dark under eye circles appear, but your skin will start to develop a dull complexion.

Product removal

Many women are guilty of going to bed with their makeup on, but it's absolutely essential that you take it off every night before bed. Not only does makeup build up in your pores, but depriving your skin of enough oxygen can cause it to dry out. It can also cause lines and wrinkles to worsen, or your skin can become red and blotchy. Your best bet is to use makeup wipes in addition to a cleanser, which not only easily removes the makeup, but deep-cleans of the junk that's built up on your face throughout the day such as dirt and pollution.

The best way to ensure your face looks its best is to develop a skin and beauty routine. It might take a few days to get used to it, but once you do, it will become habit and you'll think nothing of it. Your skin (and appearance) will thank you.

CHAPTER 15
It's in the Eyes

There really is truth to the old saying that the eyes are the windows to the soul. You can sense a lot about a person from their eyes: their confidence level, happiness, love, and more. For many women, their eyes are their favorite feature. Though for others, it is just not their favorite feature... *yet*. Maybe it's because they haven't gotten their eyes to look their absolute best. But that's about to change if you adhere to some of the following little tips and tricks.

Don't use bright colors

Leave the bright colored eyeliners and eye shadows to twenty-something's who are headed to a nightclub. Stick with subdued tones that complement your eye color to bring out the best in your eyes.

Stick to eye pencils

As you get older, liquid eyeliners can start to look harsh more than they accentuate the positive, so stick to eye pencils instead. You can also use dark shadow as eyeliner, which you can apply by using an angled makeup brush.

Throw out products once they're past their prime

Once the three year mark hits, toss the eye shadows and eyeliners and replace them. If you have been applying your eye shadow with your fingers – which you should never due as it creates a build-up of bacteria – toss them, buy new ones, and start using makeup brushes.

Use a primer

When you have creases in your eyelid and you apply eye shadow or liner, the makeup can build up and won't stay in place. Put the primer on and you can keep the makeup looking flawless and fabulous.

Use an eye cream

As you get older, fine lines can build up at the corner of your eyes, dark circles can form, and you can develop under eye circles, all of which can be combated by eye cream. Your face moisturizer doesn't count either as the skin around your eyes is extra delicate compared to the rest of your face. Look for a product that is fragrance free to reduce irritation, and keep your eye cream in the fridge so the shot of cool can reduce puffiness.

Apply the concealer correctly

When you're applying concealer, make sure to only apply it where there's discoloration rather than all over under the eye. Additionally, you should pat the makeup on, not smear it. You should also make sure to apply the concealer after the foundation and not before to blend it more evenly and allow you to use less.

Choose the right mascara

Not only should you choose mascara with the right wand, but also one that has the right formula. Look for a formula that offers you what you desire – extension, volumizing, etc. When you're applying mascara, only do so for your top lashes. Chances are you're probably still applying it to your bottom lashes. However, when you get older, applying it to the bottom can actually pull your eyes down rather than lift and open them up.

With so many different eye products out there, your best bet is to use sample products to test how your eyes respond and if you like the results before committing to full-sized products that can often be expensive. Before long, you'll find exactly what works for you.

CHAPTER 16
Love Your Lips

Many women neglect their lips, but you should always make sure to treat them right. Especially if you have a partner who you smooch regularly! Even while conversing, there are those who tend to glance at the mouth rather than the eyes, so it's even more of a reason to have your lips look their best. Adhering to the following little tips and tricks can help you do just that.

Use petroleum jelly

Apply a little petroleum jelly at night on and around your lips right before you go to sleep, and the area will be nice and hydrated when you wake up in the morning. This is especially essential to do during the winter months or when you have a cold.

Avoid dark lipsticks

Dark lipsticks can make you look older, so opt for lighter, more natural hues instead, like a complementary subtle pink color.

Use lip liner

Lip liner can not only help with the application process of the lipstick, but it can also help it stay on longer. Make sure to apply only a thin line that matches your shade of lipstick, not one that is the complete opposite (i.e. nude lipstick and brown lip liner).

Use a wrinkle fighter around your mouth

Fine lines can start to appear around your mouth as you get older, especially if you're a smoker, but using sunscreen during the day as well as a wrinkle fighter can combat the problem.

Use a lip plumper

Lips can thin as we age, and a lip plumper can make them look fuller. Sadly, not all lip-plumper's are created equal. There are many out there that make claims that they work, but don't do the job at all, so test out a bunch of them to find one that works for you.

Get teeth whitening:

Whether you get the teeth whitening done professionally or you use the at home strips, they can help your lips and the makeup look even better. There's also the added bonus of having a bright and vibrant smile that's sure to make you feel more confident and turn heads.

The skin on your lips is sensitive, so it's vital that you take extra care of the area, especially during harsh winter months when your lips can crack. Not only will you feel more beautiful by taking better care of your lips, but others are sure to notice.

CHAPTER 17
Hair, Hair, Everywhere

Hair has long been revered by many as a symbol of beauty. However, that's not actually the case. There are bald women who are stunning, women with really long hair who are beautiful, and many lengths in between. Your confidence and how you rock your 'do matter more than anything else. While most women shave their legs and underarms, let's discuss three of the other areas that you'll find hair on the body.

Hair on your head

Whether you have short hair or long, there are several things you can do to ensure that your hair looks its best and you have the ideal hair color, cut, and style for you.

Avoid blunt bangs

Blunt bangs can age you, so opt for the soft-side swept bangs instead. They can really highlight your eyes and facial features. Side swept bangs also look a lot better if they get wet, such as if you get stuck in the rain.

Forget the flat iron

Pin straight tresses can pull down your face and it especially isn't a good look if your hair is thinning, but when your hair is in curls or waves, it adds volume and makes your features look softer.

Don't sport little kid styles

Let your kids or grandkids sport the pigtails or braids while you opt for more modern styles that really bring out the best in your look.

Add some volume

Incorporating some layers can pump up the volume of your hair and really add some dimension rather than having it all one layer.

Keep it simple

Your hairstyle shouldn't be more complicated than you can manage, especially if you have a busy lifestyle. Choose one that works best for you and requires less maintenance than you're willing to devote.

Add some highlights

Highlights can add softness to your hair color and really bring out all its best aspects. Avoid doing highlights at home, especially the first time, and get them done by a professional instead.

Eyebrows

Your eyebrows may not seem like they're very important, but they can make a world of difference for the look of your face. This is why it's essential not to fool around with them too much. Adhering to a few do's and don'ts can really make the most of your look.

Elongate and arch your brows

When you let your eyebrows grow out a little at the end (lengthen, not width), and you create a slight arch, they give the illusion of pulling your eyes up and making them wider. This is an especially good technique if your eyes have gotten a bit droopy.

Don't overdo the hair removal

When your eyebrows are too thin, that can actually age you rather than make you look younger. However, they shouldn't be completely bushy either. You have to find an in-between look that works best for your face.

Stick to your natural shape

Your natural eyebrow shape is there, you just have to find it and work with it. Stray from that shape and the hair might not grow back the same as it once was.

Get them done by a professional

A reputable professional is going to be able to tweeze, wax, or pluck your eyebrows to perfection. They can see where to leave the hair alone and what shape would work best for your face.

Fill them in

To fill in voids in your eyebrows, use a powder that's a shade lighter than your brows, and use an angled brush to fill them in.

Hair down there

There are many women who question whether or not it's okay to remove the hair down there when they get older, like many do when they're younger. This is a personal choice. Whether you get a bikini wax, a little waxing, or you shave, it's about what you're comfortable with, what's easy for you to maintain, and what you like on yourself. You may also want to take your partner's opinions into consideration. But ultimately, it's your body and you have the final call.

CHAPTER 18
Going the Quick and Natural Route

Some women prefer to look like they're not wearing a stitch of makeup, while others prefer to let it show. Then there are those who *really* like to let it show by going a bit overboard. But if you're a fan of the quick and natural look, here are a few tips to get you started:

Get some sleep

Sleep is a great thing. It repairs your skin and helps prevent under eye circles all while you're grabbing a few winks.

Take care of your skin

Moisturize, exfoliate, wear sun block, and treat your skin well so you won't have to worry so much about trying to reverse the damages later.

Prime your skin

Using a primer on your skin creates that blank canvas that's essential for preventing makeup from falling into fine lines and wrinkles.

Use the right concealer and foundation

Choosing the right foundation and concealer can make your skin glow and look youthful, and once you have that, not much additional makeup is going to be necessary.

Add a little blush

Since the color in the cheeks fades as we get older, a little blush can give you that pretty rosy look that you had in your younger years.

Put on your mascara

The perfect mascara can make your eyes pop. Opt for mascara that makes others think you were just naturally born with those lashes and that they should all be jealous.

Fill in the eyebrows

Use an angled brush and powder or an eyebrow pencil to fill in the gaps and it will really enhance your eyes.

Add a touch of lip gloss or lipstick

A little bit of lip gloss and lip stick is a great finishing touch to a beautiful look.

When you're going for the natural look, you don't even necessarily have to wear eyeliner or go all out with the makeup. Sure you can do so if you'd like, but you want something that's going to get you out the door quickly while still allowing you to wear the makeup you love. Save the more dramatic makeup for the evening hours or when you have more time.

Final Thoughts

There are many who think makeup makes you beautiful, that without it you're just another "plain Jane' walking down the street. But as previously mentioned, you don't need "Top 10 flawless looks" to be considered beautiful. It is how you carry yourself, how you feel about who you are, and how you treat people. Yes, makeup is an amazing thing. By all means, have fun with it! Enhance your look, change your wardrobe, and restyle your hair. But when you feel incredible on the inside, it's really going to translate outwards. That's really what people consider true beauty.

www.ingramcontent.com/pod-product-compliance
Lightning Source LLC
Chambersburg PA
CBHW071330310526
45789CB00017B/2195